I0415278

Lecture Reprint Number 2

How To Relax
And Relieve Tension

by Bernard Jensen, D.C., N.D.,
Nutritionist

Revised and edited by Jon D. Jensen

ACKNOWLEDGEMENTS

I acknowledge and give thanks to Betty Norlin for being such a wonderful friend and for continually encouraging me and assisting me on my book writing/editing journey. Author of *"Our Bodies: The Optimal Design."* www.bettynorlin.com www.whatisholistichealth.com

I acknowledge and give thanks to Daylin Anderson, B.S. in Psychology, Cognitive and Behavioral Neuroscience/Human Development, for editing and compiling information for this lecture reprint booklet series. Daylin is a cherished friend who typed up many of these booklets for me and made it possible to finish this project. She truly is my inspiration and muse.

COPYRIGHT

Copyright @ 2019 by Jon D. Jensen

All rights reserved. No part of this book may be reproduced, stored or transmitted by any means – whether auditory, graphic, mechanical, or electronic – without written permission of both publisher and author, except in the case of brief excerpts used in critical articles and reviews. Unauthorized reproduction of any part of this work is illegal and punishable by law.

Because of the dynamic nature of the Internet, any web addresses or links contained in this book may have changed since publication and may no longer be valid.

Paperback

ISBN-13: 978-1098896942

DISCLAIMER

Any information given in this book is not intended to be taken as a replacement for medical advice. Any person with a condition requiring medical attention should consult a qualified health professional.

INTRODUCTION

My name is Jon Jensen and I have been involved in the holistic health field for many years. I have published a nutrition book, "A Simple Guide to Healthy Living" as a way to communicate with people outside my client base with information I feel is key to a healthy life. It is available on Amazon or through my website, www.jensenholistichealth.com

I've wanted to publish these health booklets for many years. My intention for editing, revising and publishing my grandfather's 21 lecture reprint booklets is rooted in my desire to continue his legacy of teaching right living through health and nutrition. Dr. Bernard Jensen spent his lifetime helping others to achieve health through education and his writing, and I feel strongly that the message is needed now more than ever.

I always marveled that my grandfather, Dr. Bernard Jensen, could write so many books and still travel, receive numerous awards, teach classes on Iridology, rejuvenation/regeneration and tissue cleansing. These lecture reprints are the product of his first lectures, typed up and stapled into booklets and originally sold for ninety-nine cents each. Thus, the beginning of a pattern where he would write and self-publish many books over his lifetime. He did end up publishing books with a couple different publishing companies, but most of his work was self-published.

DR. BERNARD JENSEN, PHD., N.D., D.C.

One of the greatest healers the world has ever known. Dr. Bernard Jensen spent over 60 years as a pioneer in the holistic health field, helping to pave the way for the alternative health revolution that we are now experiencing.

Dr. Jensen began his career at the West Coast Chiropractic College where Bernard became the youngest Chiropractor in the state of California. He traveled extensively in search of health knowledge, a search that led him to over 65 countries to observe the lifestyles of the people and their various ways of eating. Each place provided a different health secret.

Throughout his career, Dr. Jensen wrote and published over 60 books. After working with over 350,000 patients, Dr. Jensen firmly believed that nutrition is the greatest single therapy to be applied in the holistic healing arts and that "We must treat the patient, not just the disease."

Born on March 25, 1908, to parents of Danish descent, Eugen and Anna Jensen, Jorgen Bernard Jensen was raised in Stockton, California, then a small rural town in one of the richest agricultural valleys of the state. The unexpected death of his mother at age 29 from tuberculosis and consumption left three children to be raised by their father, Eugen Jensen who was a chiropractor. Very little has been written about Bernard's early life growing up in Stockton, his brother and sister, and a few comments in lectures he made about his father who was mentioned as very strict and analytical.

Early in life, young Bernard displayed the qualities needed for his future work. His penchant for being an analytical, critical, serious perfectionist blended with his sensitive, competitive, spiritual-minded personality to arm him with an unusual perspective that opened the doors to the unconventional life he was soon to enter. But before that path was firmly set, several intense learning experiences occurred which determined the direction he was to take.

Being his own worst obstacle, restless and never satisfied, he would rather study and read a book than eat or sleep. His father was a chiropractor, and young Bernard followed in his path. When he was 18 years old, Bernard entered the West Coast Chiropractic College in Oakland, California. During his four years of study, Bernard burned the midnight oil while holding down as many as two outside jobs simultaneously. The strain was immense. The capacity to push forward and the ability to persevere doggedly toward a goal were firmly established, but there was a price to pay. Bernard supported himself by working at a dairy in his spare time, and the long hours of work and study, along with poor food habits, took a heavy toll on Bernard's health. After receiving his diploma in 1929, Dr. Bernard Jensen went into practice, opening his first office in Oakland, California. He focused intently on the task of his calling which was to offer a helping hand to those suffering and in need. Dr. Bernard Jensen's devotion was complete, the hours long, his personal needs forgotten. By this time, the sacrificing of many years began to demand attention. His health began to fail. A Medical Doctor diagnosed his condition as bronchiectasis, an often-fatal lung condition, with no known cure at the time. "There is nothing I can do for you," he was told.

The young man refused to give up, searching out a Seventh Day Adventist Medical Doctor who taught him basic nutritional principles, told Dr. Bernard Jensen to leave junk food alone and promptly presented him with a maintenance program involving natural health that emphasized the return to a pure, natural and whole foods regimen. Following this program brought excellent results. Dr. Bernard Jensen was soon on the way back to health and renewed vitality. A great turning point had occurred. To be able to study nutrition and discover the laws of right living became his burning desire. Dr. Bernard Jensen turned the experience of what he learned from the Seventh Day Adventist Medical Doctor about the holistic approach into helping his patients get better and teach them how to prevent themselves from getting sick. Dr. Bernard Jensen began taking breathing exercises with Thomas Gaines, once an instructor for the New York City Police Department. Slowly, and over a period of time, his health returned, and his lungs eventually healed completely.

Using this knowledge in working with his patients the results were dramatic and effective. Dr. Bernard Jensen's attention was now riveted in this direction. Natural therapeutics became his healing mode, setting the pattern for the rest of his life. He began to travel in search of more knowledge and information.

Dr. Bernard Jensen opened his first office in Oakland, California, in 1929. He later moved to Los Angeles and expanded his practice to include branch offices at Long Beach and Santa Monica, with several chiropractors working under him. Such success had not come about overnight. In Chicago, Dr. Bernard Jensen took his post-graduate work at the National Chiropractic College and later from the Los Angeles Chiropractic College closer to home. Upon returning to California, he began an intensive study and investigation of something he was recently just learning about, the subject of iridology.

Dr. Bernard Jensen used Rocine's work as the basis for the programs used in his sanitariums-first a 25-bed sanitarium in San Leandro, California, then others in Ben Lomand and Alta Dena, and finally an 85-bed sanitarium at hidden Valley Health Ranch in Escondido, California. The sanitariums were quite successful, demonstrating the effectiveness of Rocine's ideas in working with patients. It was the Hidden Valley Health Ranch in Escondido that provided the greatest opportunity for applying the rules of right living. People in search of health and rejuvenation came to the ranch from all over the world to learn the principles that Dr. Bernard Jensen believed in, practiced, and taught.

Proper nutrition, together with sunshine, rest, exercise, fresh air and positive attitudes helped thousands of patients at Dr. Bernard Jensen's sanitariums leave behind the symptoms of chronic diseases that they have developed.

Patients came from all over the world, some to stay at his sanitariums, others for outpatient consultations and still others to attend his classes in rejuvenation and Food Studies. Thousands of New Zealanders formed clubs to follow his dietetic advice, filling out the over 350,000 people he reached, accumulated over the years. He acquired a multitude of experiences from these people individually and in group studies, acquiring information and summing it up for use in his healing work and writing.

Dr. Bernard Jensen visited the Hunza Valley, where disease, doctors, dentist and hospitals were practically nonexistent and where there were no jails, prisons or police, because there was no crime. One of Dr. Bernard Jensen's highlights of that trip was staying as a guest of the Mir of Hunza's palace for 10 days.

Dr. Bernard Jensen visited the Caucasus Mountains in the USSR to meet a 153-year-old man who had stopped riding horseback a few years earlier only because of his doctor's orders. Dr. Bernard Jensen traveled to Vilacamba, Ecuador, where heart patients were able to recuperate so marvelously. Everywhere Dr. Bernard Jensen went, he brought back some new remedy or approach to integrate into the system he taught his patients.

Dr. Bernard Jensen received his Ph.D. at the age of 75 from the University of Humanistic Studies, San Diego, California.

Dr. Bernard Jensen retired from active chiropractic practice in 1978, and devoted himself to teaching, writing and lecturing on the subjects of nutrition, rejuvenation and iridology. Around this time, Dr. Bernard Jensen completed work on a two-hour feature film, titled "World Search for Health,

Happiness and Long Life, narrated by actor Dennis Weaver.

The Academy of Science in Paris awarded Dr. Bernard Jensen a medal in 1971 for exceptional services rendered to humanity. Also, in the same year, 1971, Dr. Bernard Jensen received an honorary doctorate from the Center for the Study of Human Sciences in Lisbon, Portugal.

At a ceremony in San Remo, Italy in 1973, Dr. Bernard Jensen was presented the Ignatz Von Peczely International Iridology Gold Medal by the World Congress of Scientific Medicine, an organization embracing many medical and health disciplines.

A congress of health professionals at Aixen Provence, France, in 1974, recognized Dr. Bernard Jensen with an award for his "valuable contribution in the field of iridology."

Then in 1975, the International Naturopathic Association honored Dr. Bernard Jensen for his service to mankind through his work in the fields of health, Iridology, and nutrition.

Knighted into the Order of St. John of Malta in 1978 for his humanitarian work in the field of health, Dr. Bernard Jensen was awarded the cross of St. John at a special ceremony in New York City. This Order is the oldest chivalric organization in the world, tracing its origin back to the time preceding the first Crusade.

In 1981, at the Fifth Annual Herb Symposium, the Agnes Arber Distinguished Service award was presented to Dr. Bernard Jensen for his contributions to the current "herb renaissance."

In 1982, the National Health Federation honored Dr. Bernard Jensen with its Pioneer Doctor of the Year award at its annual convention in Long Beach, California.

In 1982, Dr. Bernard Jensen traveled to Brussels, Belgium to accept the 1982 Dag Hammarskjold award of the Pax Mundi Academy, an international organization which presents annual awards to those in the arts and sciences who have made outstanding contributions in their fields. The award, in the category of scientific merit, was for "the exceptional services rendered to collective humanity... toward international cooperation and solidarity..." Dr. Bernard Jensen was personally congratulated on his award by U. S. Ambassador, Charles Price.

In 1988 Dr. Bernard Jensen held his 80th Birthday Celebration at the Town and Country Hotel in San Diego, California, where people came from all over the world to celebrate his 80 years of life and work in the holistic health field.

In 1993 he was presented with a PhD. in natural healing arts and sciences from Westbrook University, where his iridology course was part of the school curriculum.

In 1998 and 1999 Dr. Bernard Jensen received awards from the IIPA for his work in iridology.

In 2000 Dr. Bernard Jensen was awarded by Nature Sunshine an honorary award for his outstanding contributions to iridology and herbology before five thousand people.

On February 22, 2001 a month before his 93rd birthday, Dr. Bernard Jensen passed away at 92 years old.

The short biography above about Dr. Bernard Jensen is a small part of a larger biography I am writing about my grandfather's life. If you are interested in learning more I will be blogging and have more information at www.bernardjensen.org

In the 21 lecture reprint booklets you'll see products or foods that might not be commonly found today. I left some things in to give the flavor of that time period and what he was thinking at that time. I also left in quotes or sayings from that era. I edited misspellings and grammatical errors. But overall, I feel that these booklets give down to earth advice and can still be regarded as basic knowledge in the mainstream health field today. A lot of his products are no longer available, but you can find what remains on my website, www.jensenholistichealth.com

I hope you enjoy these lecture reprint booklets as much as I do and take them for what they are. If nothing else, a novelty and glimpse of the past. A simple approach of one of the early promoters of healthy living. Alongside such greats of that era like Paul Bragg, Jack LaLanne, Dr. Max Gerson, V.E. Irons and Dr. Bronner at the beginning of a health revolution.

Jon D. Jensen

HOW TO RELAX AND RELIEVE TENSION

"My purpose is to serve and I must serve my purpose."

Bernard Jensen, Ph.D., D.C., N.D.

What is relaxation? Relaxation is the action of unbinding, or unbending the mind from severe application or tension, releasing it from ordinary occupation or care. It is a recreation and rest needed for loosening or slackening of the tense muscle and nerve fibers. It is a release from intensity, a diminution of vigor and extreme energies.

Most of us are in severe application all the time. It is not enough to tell you to "go home and forget it." You will go home and may seem to forget it, but you merely bury it in the subconscious only to have the difficulty rise again and torment you. The thing to do is RELAX, and relaxation, as I see it, is a mental thing, a matter of education of the body through the mind.

First, visualize relaxation; reach for it; gesture for it; feel it, until finally, it becomes a part of you. We know that our habits can be either good or bad and relaxation is the best habit of all. If we can make a habit of relaxation, through a hobby, through association with good companions, through doing something different in our daily lives, then relaxation will come naturally.

If relaxation has to be forced upon you, by being told to, "go to a show" and you go to a show whether you want to or not, it is possible that you will not relax. Relaxation comes when you do the things you want to do. If they are things you love to do, so much the better.

Relaxation is much talked about today, and I find in my practice, that we are moving in an entirely different direction from that I was taught in college. There are so many people coming into my office with troubles we did not hear about years ago.

Formerly, we looked for displacements in the body, twists, a vertebra out of place, high blood pressure, diabetes, arthritis or nephritis, and we made all kinds of tests. After the diagnosis we had a set treatment. This was the set procedure then, but today we are taking another direction. We deal with body habits and thinking processes. This is an important step in diagnosing.

Relaxation is one of the many things we must consider in our health program, along with food, exercise, sunshine, water, and the main things that go to make up a good health program. Invariably, we realize that relaxation is something most of us miss. There are very few people who have ever experienced real health, so they do not know what it is. We are hoping, therefore, in this message, to enable you to touch, experience, or to arrive at a place where you are aware that there is such a thing as relaxation.

There are very few people who ever feel wonderful mentally and physically, so they have no idea what it is. You will never have an inspiration nor attain complete happiness unless you do feel wonderful, so let us try to feel and experience what relaxation is, as it plays a big part in attaining complete health.

Let us find out what it is to feel wonderful, for once, and then strive to get hold of it. After a while it will become automatic for you to relax whenever you feel the need or want to. I believe this is the secret of my being able to work as I do. In a matter of a few moments I can relax and let go so completely that I can pick up and go on for hours, again and again. I feel I know the extreme in relaxation just as I know the extreme in tension while working.

There comes a time in our lives when we must take inventory to find out just what our assets are and add up the good in our lives so that we know just exactly what we are doing in life that is really worthwhile.

I know many of us look at ourselves and say, "I am not accomplishing anything." To that person who wants to accomplish I say, "If you cannot accomplish, you are indeed miserable and you are unable to relax." That person who does not wish to accomplish anything or who can accomplish anything he wants to in one hour a day and relax the rest of the day, does not need my suggestions.

We must take an inventory of ourselves, look inside and find out what kind of individuals we are; find out where the happiness for each lie; what we must do in order to become right with ourselves.

Most of us are all tied up in knots. Our stomachs are tied up like Chinese feet and we are snappy, hypercritical, over-anxious and often too ambitious. These things bring on tensions in the body. Some people think tension is created by doing the wrong thing but that is not always the case. We can do too much of the right thing and this too brings on tension, for it wears out the chemical elements that have been overworked.

Some say, "I can't relax." We cannot relax because relaxing is an educational process. It may take a year for you to educate yourselves to sleep properly and peacefully with consequent rest. But remember, you have probably spent five years breaking down your mental philosophy to the place where you simply cannot sleep relaxed.

You must learn to rest the mind. To sleep with a mind in turmoil means you will not rest and you will wake up tired. The rested mind is worth more than a sleeping mind. The energy and effort we put into trying to sleep could be spent in beautiful thoughts or thankfulness, for instance, for without thankfulness we cannot relax.

Look at everything in a joyful state of mind. Dismiss negative things, bless things. If you learn these things, you have learned much. If you learn to bless things, you have learned the biggest lesson. To bless a thing is to dismiss it. To bless an irritation, you dismiss that irritation. If you do not dismiss everything irritating, with a blessing, these irritations will hang upon you until you do.

WHY THE NEED OF RELAXATION?

We are moving into a new era, a high-pressure era, a mental and psychic era. It is not uncommon to have a patient come to me and say, "I am nervous, unstrung, high strung, and I have the fidgets so that I cannot concentrate. "I find that he has been going to all kinds of doctors and the doctors have been testing him for blood pressures, looking for thyroid trouble or diabetes. This trouble was created in his mind by his actions and reactions in the things he did or did not do.

Do not wait until you have trouble and then go to a doctor. A great deal can be done in the prevention of your troubles if you will just sit down and think things out.

Mental tension can be relayed to any part of the body. That which was once an internal expression finally becomes an external one by developing into some physical ailment of the body. Physically, it works out through the different muscles.

Eighty percent of the body structure consists of muscles, and twenty percent of bone. Play or action, brought forth in the muscles, had its origin in the nervous system. Our thinking controls all direction in the body and is reflected in the nervous system and most of the tension in the body comes from our thinking. Muscles are connected with nerves that lead to the spine and when you raise your arm many muscles are brought into play, but before this action can take place, a message must go from the brain centers through the thinking processes to the muscles. If you cut the nerves the muscles can no longer work.

Through tension we produce cramps in the bowels. Tense muscles are responsible for many of our diseases such as colitis, goiter, diabetes, heart trouble, nephritis and arthritis. Remember, we are talking about relaxing.

It is not possible to live without tone in our muscles, but it is the excess and the constant over-tone that is the breakdown influence. Over-activity of muscles produces acids. Over-activity of nerves produces acid. Brain cells can break down under too much thinking. Although brain cells can be rebuilt at the rate of two per second, when we tear down three cells or more per second, we get into trouble; we have a toxic state of affairs and a chemical shortage sets in. Irritation sets up in the nerves and muscles when there is over-activity and excessive contraction.

Your state of health may not come from present over-use but from past over-use. Many people have lost nerve force and cannot secure the proper body response. Then it becomes a matter of re-education of the mind; a matter of establishing a new system of thinking. It is a matter of properly feeding the worn-out cell life and of learning everything we can for the recuperation of the body.

The remedy, and my work, is to start at the beginning and get at the cause of the trouble. When you tell me you have high blood pressure I want to know what you are thinking. Nine times out of ten, high blood pressure comes from what you think and not what you do. Many other troubles come from our thinking and not from physical action.

The glands are affected by every thought. We have gland specialists trying to take care of the thyroid glands, when in most cases, the trouble is the result of wrong thinking.

We cannot set aside diet and work twenty-four hours a day and say, "Well, my thoughts are right so I will be all right". If you do not take care of your body, both mentally and physically, it will go back to where it came from; back to the "dust of the earth."

Play is one thing we neglect most as we grow older, and relaxation is found in play. We must work, but we must also play. As a matter of fact, anything which produces relaxation becomes play.

Ninety-five percent of acids in the body are manufactured through lack of relaxation which means a toxic condition brought on by improper thyroid action. People reach a point where they seem unable to control their thoughts or their bodies and they become "thyroid-sick." Practically everyone, I dare say, who jumped off "suicide bridge" in Pasadena, Califomia, suffered poor health. They had thyroid glands which bothered them and threw them "off balance."

The Thyroid gland is largely controlled by our mental attitude. We must not, therefore, abuse this or any other gland by wrong thinking and tension. Calm, relaxation, and peace will relax the thyroid gland more than anything else. We all have so many troubles today and so many tense thoughts that get a grip on us. We are so serious about everything! But remember, there is nothing so bad that it could not be worse.

Work can be a hardship, or it can be relaxing. There are many people killing themselves through what they make of their work. There are those who find relaxation in their work but who drive the body beyond what it should be called upon to do. Eight hours of work is usually sufficient for any one person, even in work you love to do. To go beyond that creates the opposite of relaxation, or tension; while four hours of work that we do not want to do, through resentment and resistance, can exert enough influence to eventually kill you.

Sixteen hours of work you love to do, probably would not hurt for the time being and may be carried on for years, but sixteen hours of work will wear out the minerals of the body faster than they can be replaced by the digestive system. We can only put so many minerals into the body and it takes so many hours to use them up, so many hours to recuperate. Thus, we find that there is no time left for rest or relaxation.

As for those of us who live in the city, think of the noise of the radio and the wrangling sounds that come over the air, the clang of street cars, fire responses, ambulances and other street noises. The "fear" posters like, "Cancer. One in eight has it. You may be next!" Constant irritation from the all-day long exposures to excitation is the cause of many nervous breakdowns.

On the job we are in a rush. At five o'clock the stenographer is rushing to get through, trying to get as many words written as possible. At quitting time there is a crush of crowds, people hurrying to get home on street cars, automobiles and buses, while newsboys run in and out of traffic screaming exciting headlines. A man may, for a time, own his own business, but the business soon owns him. This is City Life! A constant bustle and commotion! On the other hand, a relaxed body, walking across the busy streets of Los Angeles, New York City, or any other big city, will really invite trouble, will it not?

These distractions all have their effect on the body. We respond to these distractions and our bodies become tense, like a taut wire. The physical body cannot follow the "fast train" of thoughts which has been worked out by civilization today. The human frame eventually breaks under such a load. Some seem to get used to it but most of us are overcome.

The challenge of time, must be met. The pressure of "getting something out by five o'clock," means that the average stenographer does not know how to relax. The average executive takes baths and massages once or twice a week, so that he can relax. Mother goes downtown with her child and has to "buck" the traffic and the people in the stores and comes home a "wreck". The husband on his job has not been getting along with the boss; the job irks him and he feels like a misfit and wishes he was someone else or somewhere else. Mother and father, together at night, are no example for their children because their minds are not relaxed, and the children, as a result become irritable, and we have a whole family disunited and made unhappy because of the irritation.

How are we going to remedy this? What are we going to do about the blood pressures that are so high, resulting from these irritations? What are we going to do about the glands which have been pinched because we have not enough money to carry out the plans we would like to and to do all the things we want to do? What are we going to do about these "twists" in our bodies which come from muscles strained and from tension on one side of the body more than on the other?

Is it our love problem we are going to straighten out? Is it our money problems? How are we going to get to the bottom of these things? Perhaps it will take just a good laugh. Sometimes a good laugh will do more for us than anything else. Do we laugh enough? Do we see the bright side of things? Shall we continue going through life like a high-strung bow that eventually breaks? What suggestions can we possibly make? Do we just say, "forget it?" What are you going to do? Are you going to have an understanding of them? Or are you going ahead and just let things skip by and bear it? Can things be changed? It may be worth a try. I suggest that we do try and see what can come out of it all.

WHAT TO DO ABOUT IT

Let us realize that we need time out for relaxation. Let us get the "feel" of relaxation. We must do this in order to balance the fight against daily activities and wrong thinking. We must recognize through progressive right thinking, progressive right living, progressive right exercises, relaxation exercises that we can learn to relax. Recognize the need for a relaxed body and mind. Ease of mind begets ease of body.

The person who is under high tension finds it difficult to relax. Relaxation is a thing to be cultivated. You cannot learn it in one night. You cannot read about it and know all about it in one day. You must take time out to study and try to realize what is going on and what is to be done.

Relaxation is just as important to your body as putting food into your stomach. As food nourishes you, relaxation comforts and soothes your tired mind; releases your tight muscle strings so that new blood can flow easily and recuperation and regeneration of cell life can take place.

Your body is a valuable asset only when it is working at your command. Realize that you own this body. The ownership of anything is as good as the use you have out of it, whether it be money, occupational tools, or your body. Your body is your tool in trade. No job can be completed well when it is done under continuous tension, for as we said, it is the too tight bow that breaks.

The life within you determines what kind of a job shall be done through your body tissues. That which is deep within your body, mentally and spiritually, is what makes the external world you live in. The same causes and effects existing in the world exists also in our body. The tension in the world today existed first in human beings. Can you imagine that this war, or any war, would be the result of a peaceful relaxation? No! Tension is the expression of human minds and bodies and that is where the first care and education should be, in the mind of man. There are very few people who will take care of their bodies and work for their higher good, but we will not have peace of mind nor peace on earth until we do. Expressions today are uncontrolled, automatic and this comes mostly from the high-tensioned living.

When you walk at night and look into the sky, is there anything there that excites you so that the whole body becomes tense? There is relaxation in watching a sunrise; this does not drive you to distraction, does it? But, does the crowing of a rooster distract you? How about the green of a pasture? Here is relaxation and peace for a tired soul; this would give release from a city-created tension!

Relax and let go. The finest sensations we have are when we sit down and relax. Go into the animal world and watch the deer and the fawns. As soon as a little noise is heard, they become tense and alert and off they dart. Noises that are not of nature can be most disturbing.

When we get close to nature we have a perfectly relaxed body. As we breathe the air we recognize that something must come from it that is good. We must get fresh air; if possible, air which comes from and through places where there are many trees, for trees oxygenate the air. People go to places in Georgia or Michigan, for instance, to be among the pine trees which throw off a lot of ozone, the health-giving property.

When we get close to nature we have a perfectly relaxed body, truly, for we become one with nature and attach ourselves to the situation that is best for our bodies' welfare. We can have bodies capable of working to capacity at any time, but not if we break them down by using them continually beyond capacity.

I repeat, relax and let go. The finest sensations we have are when we sit down and relax. Just consideration is not being given to the troubles we are having today. It is high time we do something about it.

Perhaps you have heard me tell the story about my son David. One day when he was four years old, he was pushing a boat around in a fishpond in front of the sanitarium and I was afraid he was going to fall in. David said he would be careful and he knew he would be all right. I wanted to push him in so that he would have the experience, but I did not. I walked away and in a few moments heard the inevitable splash. I did not know whether to say, "I told you so," or to spank him. I did nothing.

That night David was cutting out pictures with a razor blade and I told him he should use a pair of scissors as they were not as dangerous. I said, "David, this morning I told you that you would fall into the fishpond and what happened?" He replied, "I fell in." I went on, "and tonight, I tell you not to use a razor blade because you might cut yourself, but to use a pair of scissors instead. You tell me you will not cut yourself. It could happen, you know. Tell me, what do you use your brains for?" Quick as a flash, he replied, "I use my brains to forget with."

There is a situation to think about. This mental faculty of memory is difficult to control and brings us pictures of the past to stare at and thus spoil our present moments. We do not have the faculty of forgetting and so remember everything. Every experience has left its mark in every cell and muscle in our bodies. So, it behooves us all to develop a philosophy which allows a relaxed outlook no matter what happens. Telling you to go home and forget it is not a cure for your problem. We are going to have to try out a new attitude. This will be an education.

When we stop to think about all the books being written and sold today, we notice the "best sellers" carry titles such as, "Peace Within," "Peace with the Soul," "Relaxation," "Flight from the City," "Get Rid of that Nerve Tension." These are the subjects which seem to be in demand. There must be a reason for writing them and there must be a reason for people seeking relaxation in the reading of them. Rather than just talk about relaxation, let us deal more with causes.

I am wondering if it is not possible to wake up wisely in the morning. I wonder if it is not possible to be more of an optimist than a pessimist. I am wondering if it is possible to rest a few moments before eating, so there would be no need for a tense body. Is it possible to ensure a good night's sleep by ironing out your troubles before you go to bed? It would mean going to bed relaxed instead of under tension. Is it possible for us to convert ourselves and change some of our habits of having, so that relaxation will be an automatic thing in our lives, rather than a thing to anxiously work out? This "anxiety" and this "trying" to work out relaxing is in itself a tension-creating thing.

I know a man who had a nervous breakdown because he had not taken care of himself; he had not relaxed or let go as he should have done. A doctor advised him to take a two-year rest. This man was the manager of a big concern and so he replied, "That is impossible. How can I take a rest? What are they going to do without me? How can they get along?" To which the doctor replied, "Keep on working for a few more weeks and they will have to do without you entirely! You must take a rest." The man decided to follow the doctor's advice and take a rest. During the two years' time he travelled all over the world and toward the latter part of the time he felt he just could not wait until he reached home. He felt such anxiety concerning his job he could scarcely wait to get back. When he walked into his office he found the man hired to carry on his work of management sitting in his easy chair, his feet up on the desk, reading a funny paper! Well, this man could not understand. He had never had time to read the funny paper or to put his feet up on his desk; he exclaimed, "What's the idea? How do you ever get time to read the funny paper and sit back with your feet on the desk?" The reply was, "You had to be sent away on account of your health, so I decided to keep my health and relax a little now and then. That's the reason I take a break. I don't want to make your mistake."

THE ART OF RELAXATION

Bear in mind that eighty percent of your body is involved in muscle and nerve control. One of your best-informed doctors on muscle control, Dr. DeJamette, tells us that all diseases are caused from "twists" in the body. That may seem to be an unusual statement, but when you have appendicitis you have greater contraction on one side than on the other. Every disease seems to carry a "twist" with it.

A short time ago there was a book published by Eastman Kodak Company in which one of the illustrations was of a spinal column; another, that of the person afflicted with tuberculosis. It showed the upper part of the spine to be tubercular with a lesion in the lung. A doctor was treating that lesion, but we noted in the picture of the spine, behind the lung, a tremendous curve right behind the lesion, the twist or pull leading to the lung.

Emotional shock can cause a "twist" in the spine and this can cause a pressure in certain muscle structures of the body. Interference with the proper nerve supply leading to the spine develops bronchitis, pleurisy, or any disease of the lung, even tuberculosis.

Many people come to me for adjustment. I formerly put them on a table and started right to work on them. Sometimes I would find muscles of the neck tense and as I began to work over these muscles, I would find out that the person had money troubles. The money troubles had settled in the neck. Sometimes it was husband and wife trouble that got them "in the neck", or occupational trouble.

Sometimes a patient had been so serious about everything that he did not know what it was to relax. One can concentrate too intensely.

Our college yells in nearly every state have something to say about, "Give it to them in the neck!" The neck feels and registers all tensions in the body first. A relaxed person has a very limber neck. To adjust these tensions or release them, we adjust the neck, re-aligning the vertebra, but to endeavor to do this without first adjusting the mind, would be the same as not treating a patient at all. "First things must come first," for the good book says: "Be thou not stiff-necked." When I find a stiff neck, I know that the possessor of it must either indulge in a good cry or talk it out. We must get to the source of the trouble. When I say "talk it out" I MEAN talk it out. Anything of a disturbing nature which you keep in your mind, is as bad as any physical disturbance. You will get along better if you "get it off your chest." Do not think that imagination, fear, and such things, are not real. They are very real as long as you hold onto them. They are definitely things that should be removed.

Speaking of talking things out, it is just as necessary to share the good things as to share or talk about the "irritating things" in life. Any time you hold a secret that would be good for someone else to know, there will be trouble for you instead of joy. Share the good you know with someone else.

I spoke before about the importance of the doctor knowing the cause of the patients' troubles. For an example, a lady came into my office suffering from colitis. I immediately began a study of her background.

What did she have in her make-up that had become involved in this colitis? Colitis, you know, is inflammation of the large intestine, and is very painful. "I cannot sleep," is always a complaint of the colitis sufferer, and it is not a matter of food alone. I treated her mind and her colitis disappeared. This patient had gone to ten or fifteen doctors for relief and had tried all kinds of diet before coming to me. I do not wish to criticize other doctors' routines, but I always treat the mental right along with the physical.

Unless your mind is at ease and the muscles all over the body are at ease, you will not rid yourself of your trouble. Ulcers of the stomach follow the same pattern as colitis. The Mayo brothers say that ninety percent of the stomach ulcers have their origin in love or money troubles. Fretting and worrying are contributing causes to this trouble. Many times, I know I can clear away the trouble in a man if I can get the woman of the house to help out, but when the woman is working out of the home and the couple live on a coffee and doughnut diet, we do not get very far.

We often speak of "mind over matter" and believe me. Mind comes first. Remember, a good healthy life comes from mental and spiritual uprightness. That is righteousness. We do not want to think it is only a matter of bones and muscles. We measure up to and react to that which is in our minds. We injure or build our bodies with our minds.

A great deal of trouble may be caused by a diaphragm which is not relaxed, and the diaphragm is a very important part of the body. It is the midriff which divides the chest from the abdomen and must be kept strong. A good hearty laugh works this diaphragm up and down; deep breathing works it up and down, or in and out, as you wish, and this will bring on relaxation. Your lungs are literally gasping for breath when you sigh.

The function of the diaphragm is one of the most important functions of the body. Through its action it keeps the abdominal organs moving, and when that diaphragm becomes tight, the other organs become tight also. There is a fluid known as peritoneal, which flows between all the organs and if the diaphragm is not working properly, this fluid is not able to flow as it should. This causes acids to accumulate and these accumulated acids cause contraction and adhesions develop. The most delightful way to exercise the diaphragm is to laugh. In show business there is a type of actor who feels his work is successful when he can convulse his audience into 'belly laughs', not an elegant expression but, believe me, a good healthy performance for all concerned. We do not indulge enough in good heart-warming laughs. There was a time when a hearty laugh was considered ill-bred. Now, we are too serious, too busy thinking and looking at the wrong side of the picture; yet, nothing is so serious we cannot relax and see the funny side of a situation. This is necessary if we are to keep our balance. Scan the advertising section occasionally and note what is wanted. I read an ad the other day which stated, "Wanted: Piano, on terms with mahogany legs." Read the personal columns for laughs.

A young lady came to see me one day and while talking to me she remarked that she could not seem to see a joke in anything; she could not see anything funny to laugh at. This is a pitiful state in which to be. I did not think of it at the time of the interview; too intense myself, I guess, but in going over her case in my mind, I recalled that she had said, "I've had my teeth taken out and a stove moved in." I must admit that she gave me one of the best laughs I have had in many a day.

It takes six muscles to make a smile and 120 to make a frown, so for economy's sake, let us use only the six muscles and spare ourselves the lines and wrinkles.

If you have prolonged work to do, stop at intervals and relax. Do not drive an automobile for four or five hours at a time. Stop and stretch your legs; take a few deep breaths; exercise a little. If you are a stenographer and work all day, pounding out many words a minute, stop every hour and give your body a chance to relax. Relaxing means becoming limp and motionless. Make a business of it. Nerves must carry messages, but they must also have a time to become inactive and at ease, or disease will result.

Marconi, said that he would work out the radio wave system we have today, and he did. He knew that everybody had been working on the principle that radio waves would have to work through resistance, but Marconi could not, and did not, see a "resistance program" in his mind. Have we not been trying to follow others in trying to find a way to relax, when we must find it in our own way? We follow doctors who are "resisting, combating, and fighting" disease; who treat disease without changing conditions that cause the disease. A non-resistance program would bring considerable relief and relaxation by recognizing we are one with the Creative Power. We do not have to recognize things in life, such as disease, ill health or poverty. We can live so that we use all emotion for ease, ill health or poverty. We can live so that we use all emotion for good. You can fight, you can war on things, you can "buck" and resent and have a resistance program on your hands, but the Point is, you can also "let go".

SLEEP KNITS THE RAVELED SLEEVE OF CARE

It is not necessary to sleep, but IT IS NECESSARY TO REST. Most people want to sleep because of the state of mind they find themselves in. I sincerely believe that if a person could absolutely rest his mind, could make this mind an absolute blank for one hour a day, he would not need sleep. He could derive as much benefit in that one hour as he could derive in twenty-four hours of sleep. I do not believe; however, a man can do this today. I am pointing out the extreme toward which one might work.

The person who goes to bed saying: "I will not go to sleep tonight," does not recognize that the subconscious mind cannot take a joke and so will not according to the instruction. He gets the result; he does not sleep. Suggestion is very important in keeping yourself relaxed. The suggestions you give yourself before you go to sleep will determine the kind of rest you have.

You may go to bed disgusted, discouraged; the day has been a "blue" one; you want to get it over with and forget it. If you relax when you lie down and rest, that would be much more important than the sleep you might get. If you sleep fifteen hours twisting and turning, that sleep will do you no good. In the morning you should wake up and feel rested enough to want to work. Some people can become rested with two or three hours of sleep. Rest comes only when you give yourself the proper suggestion, as: "relax and let go."

Suggestions made at night follow you all through your sleeping hours. I have seen more than one case of bed-wetting cured by the suggestion made to the child before going to sleep that, "If there is an urge to urinate, awaken immediately and get up." You can tell a child, after he is asleep, to turn over and if you do it strongly and firmly enough, you will see him turn over.

When you go to bed at night, you do not want to think about food and acid conditions. You want to think about creating an alkaline condition, if you think about conditions at all. So, if suggestions are going to follow you throughout the night, you might as well have those which come from a pleasant mind instead of one from an acid disposition. The acid condition or disposition will produce a physical condition which your sleeping hours will have to take care of and your sleeping hours should be recuperative. Why add over-work? Pessimism, "blues," resentment, resistance, hate, jealousy, anxiety, all are created in an acid-producing mind.

I know that a lot of us cannot wait until we change our minds or until we actually get this thing working for us, so I have put together an exercise. It is possible to get the body and the mind to go in the right direction but in order to do so we have to build up a good circulation. We must get new blood to circulate and we do it with the right physical exercise and food. In the meantime, while we are waiting for our minds to take on different ideas, let us make some, suggestions to ourselves. Here is one of the best ways to make a suggestion to yourself: Count seven, three times, say to your mind, "When I count to seven and then get to number seven in my mind, I am going to feel drowsy. I am going to sleep; I am going to feel peaceful; everything is in harmony; I have finished this day well; I have done all that I can. I ask to be strengthened for tomorrow in order to carry on and finish up that which was not finished today. I ask that I may carry on well with my work tomorrow. I ask that my strength go into recession for absolute peace. I ask that all power and energy go into absolute recession, so that there is no more activity mentally or physically." Suggest to yourself that you are a child of God; that you are in good hands, the hands of God; that you will be well taken care of.

Then start counting, looking always toward the number seven in order to give you that complete drowsiness that you seek. Then start counting with the idea of one being the most important number; then two being less important. You can see number three less. Number four is getting less and less. You come to number five and if you hardly see the number five, you are getting drowsier, so that you can scarcely see the number six. With number seven, you are still drowsier and I am sure it will not be long before you are sound asleep.

If you are not asleep, start over again; "Number one, I am getting drowsy; I am getting ready for a good sleep. Number two, I am getting drowsier. Sleep is coming upon me. "When you come to seven, you come to the natural number of universal peace and so, carry on and count those numbers to seven. If you have to count four, five, or six or seven times, all right, just keep counting to seven, always knowing that when you come to seven, there is a more complete rest coming to you than ever before. You will not pass many sevens before you will go into complete slumber.

"WHAT FOOLS THESE MORTALS BE, TO PUT INTO THEIR MOUTHS THAT WHICH POISONS THE MIND"

What about the food you eat in relation to relaxation? Warm food brings on relaxation. If you are in need of relaxation it is a sign that you need, among other things, lecithin and Vitamin B. When I point out that you need certain things, they are specific. On the other hand, if we eat natural foods we would not need the specific things. This is something you should leave to your doctor. You cannot say that you will live in the sun and "eat anything" in the way of food, take coffee and doughnuts any time you like, and get away with it. You must learn about yourself and everything that is involved in your living and live according to Nature's law to the best of your ability. You reap the results of your living habits.

Specific chemical elements we need are phosphorus, manganese, iodine and sulphur. They are the crude, coarse elements; the brain and nerve elements. The "trace" elements are very necessary also and are found best in the fish and sea foods. Pineapple and egg yolk have a lot of iodine in them, also phosphorus and lecithin. There is sulphur in onions, cabbage, cauliflower, broccoli, and these all help drive the oils and nerve fats to the brain. It might be a good thing to have a sulphur vegetables when you have protein, for all proteins are brain and nerve foods.

Missouri Black Walnuts are very high in manganese and can be used in your nut loaves, liquefied drinks and nut butters. A good brain and nerve cocktail can be made with black cherry juice, pineapple juice and egg yolk. Add one-half teaspoon of powdered Nova Scotia dulse and one tablespoon of wheat germ for Vitamin E value.

When you break down the nerve system you also deteriorate the glandular system so food for the nerves also helps the glands. Proteins are a wonderful brain and nerve food, but even though they help overcome the effects which fear has produced, they will not remove the fear. The best way to prevent fear, from breaking us down is to not allow fear to enter into our mind. Food is one of the main things to be considered in getting good relaxation. Ulcers of the stomach are produced from foods and ulcers certainly are not conducive to relaxation. A revolution going on in the form of a disease, anywhere in the body, is not going to allow us to sit down and enjoy any beautiful music which may come over the radio or phonograph or through anyone who is playing it for our entertainment.

We must have freedom of action in all parts of our body and freedom from pain above all things. We must recognize that there is a way to live and a way to put all of this together. There is a health program which takes in everything in nature. Many books written today are written by doctors who want us to know more about relaxation.

We cannot tell a person to relax, then let him live on coffee and doughnuts, or their equivalent, and have him all tied up with constipation or headaches and expect him to believe that relaxation will come from his mental processes only. You cannot "eat just anything," and expect to relax. If you have colitis you must be careful of raw foods. If you have irritation of the bowel, or a stomach irritation, you must be careful of certain acids.

A little lady who had returned to the sanitarium, was telling me that she was working in a home where she had to eat everything. It tasted very nice and she thought, "Oh, I can eat it now," and did, enjoying it tremendously, so far as taste is concerned. She prayed that it would not do anything harmful to her body. She is back at the sanitarium now and has a bursitis, and an arthritic settlement, in her shoulder. True, she prayed about it, but prayers are not answered when we do not do the right thing. We cannot expect the right, when we do the wrong.

Few doctors consider the importance of relaxation when it comes to releasing acids which cause irritation or tension in the muscle structure of the body. One of the main things to consider is that harmony is a state of relaxation. Discord or inharmony destroys; inharmony develops disease.

There are foods prepared with the use of coal tar products. Coal tar acts as a definite irritation in the body. Coal tar is found in the coloring of butter and in

preservatives, condiments and the bleaches used in white flour. Coal tar can absolutely cause allergies in the body. Many people have colds produced through coal tar irritations in the body. Such food as catsup causes irritation to the body because of the use of baking soda in its formula. Many of our foods are sweetened with baking soda. At one time I worked in a creamery where we took sour cream. Ice cream is sold as an "end product," which is brought about through an excess of milk in our creameries. Sometimes, the worst products are made into foods we eat, especially if it takes coal tar preservatives or baking soda to sweeten them. Many people are suffering from diabetes and cannot take certain sweets and they resort to saccharin, which is 400 times sweeter than sugar, but it is made out of coal tar, and in time, its use causes irritation in the body.

Cooking in certain metal vessels that erode into the food as it is being cooked in them, in time, can act as an irritant to the body, which is the reason so many doctors today are opposed to the metal vessels that are being used. Such irritation in the stomach will eventually produce ulcers and other diseases that we fall heir to.

Remember too, the fluids which go into your body should not be the kind that will break down the kidneys. Drinks that are irritating to the body, such as alcoholic drinks, coca cola or the soft drinks which so many people drink today, produce irritations which finally cause tensions. So then, all our talk about relaxation will do no good under such conditions, for there is a tightness and a tension set up in the body, which is often caused from irritations produced from the use of these bad drinks and foods.

Colors, too, have their effects in tension or relaxation. Red, for instance, is most irritating to some, invigorating to others. Blue and green are relaxing. In the spring, everything is green and from this God-given color you get relaxation which you can get from nothing else.

Clothes can form an irritant to some of us. Some like certain suits or dresses, and enjoy wearing them, but other clothes, which have come to them under unpleasant circumstances, irritate them and they cannot stand to wear them. This is a form of irritation in the mind. It is necessary for us to realize that we must, whenever possible, remove all irritations in life in order to gain relaxation.

About five years ago we took 20 people up to Mt. Hollywood. Most of them were over sixty and declared they could not walk more than a block in town, yet they walked the three-mile hike up Mt. Hollywood. It is not work which kills people; it is the tension created. It is not the work which is hard; it is the tension involved. Before completing your task, where there is tension, you are tired out.

Through certain baths you may become relaxed. Pine needle baths and Epsom salts baths are relaxing. Idly swinging in a hammock will be surprisingly relaxing. Every running brook has its possibilities for relaxing. Did you ever try sleeping beside one? It is wonderful! Lindlahr wrapped patients in cold sheets and covered them with blankets; they grew warm and relaxed.

Social relations must be taken into consideration when seeking relaxation. Some people can relax with people around them while others are irritated. If you find you have a job, where you are working with people and that you get "fed up" with people, then your relaxation should be where there are no people, or your hobby should be one where you can get away from people. Those who work in such jobs like bookkeeping, or with metals, rocks or machinery, and if they love people, then their hobby should be one where they will be with people and so balance the day. Thus, social relationships should be considered in the seeking of relaxation.

There has been a question about "suggestions" in the mornings. Let me say that suggestion is the most powerful thing in the world. Suggestions come to us through images held before our minds. If the image out shadows or out pictures everything else we can see, we accept that as the real thing. If we say, "I just know I am not going to sleep tonight." You will not sleep under ordinary peaceful conditions. If you do sleep after such expression, you only sleep because of utter exhaustion, for the sub-conscious mind is powerful enough to keep before you the image you created, "I will not sleep."

In order to allow that sleep center to hold away or to become the greatest image of your life, it must have expression. You have expressed to yourself, "I will not sleep," and if that is the most powerful thing, and is out shadowing and out picturing all else, you will do just what your subconscious mind has been told to do in your suggestion.

This can be carried on and on, and when you say, "what I feared has come upon me," you are expressing this truth. So, let us see to it that what we suggest to ourselves is that which we really wish. If you talk success to yourself, you will be successful, but it you prove to yourself that you are a failure and so express yourself, you cannot be a success. The words "I am" are the most powerful words ever uttered. There is no such thing as being a success and a failure at the same time or being "blue" and "happy" at the same time, nor loving and hating at the same time. You must take whatever suggestion is before you and live it. Live every suggestion that comes to you.

When the suggestion, "things are not so good," come to you, it may be that things are better than you think. There is a possibility that with all the pessimistic things we hear today, optimism could take its place.

Optimism is a health-building proposition and to start the day with the knowledge that you have a hard day to get through, and you say, "I do not know how I am going to make it," you are looking for trouble. You are suggesting trouble. You are living trouble before you even get there. Many of us are "living trouble"; we are not living life. So, I say this, if it is difficult to take on a whole day at a time, think of what one little lady said to me once:

"Life by the inch, is a cinch; Life by the yard, can be very hard".

WITH ALL THY GETTING, GET UNDERSTANDING

Gossip wears out a lot of nerve energy; just the opposite of relaxation. Three-fourths of the thoughts we entertain and the things we hear, should never have come to our attention. All experiences are good when we use them for good. All experiences are bad if you use them that way. You must develop a good philosophy of Life.

Be honest with yourself; do not work against yourself. Sit quietly; go into the silence within yourself. Clear all distracting things out of your mind and body and just see how wonderful you can feel. Think only of good for yourself, your children, your neighbors, and thus free yourself. This freedom will bring relaxation. If you want this freedom, you must have a spiritual philosophy as well as a mental philosophy.

Remember, we are all different so make allowances for this fact. Did you ever sit in a bus or a streetcar and take note of the many faces you see? No two are alike; each one is different, reflecting different characteristics. We are all products of creation. We cannot help what faces have been given us, but we can help what we make of them, as we all realize that what we think and what we eat leaves an imprint upon our faces. Never make comparisons or pass judgment.

It is not good for one who is fashionably dressed and looks well physically, to ask another why he does not look as well; we should never ask this question, even in our thoughts, for thoughts are things. Some people are born with certain qualities and few limitations, while others are born with limitations as to health, looks and conditions over which they apparently had no control. Therefore, we must not expect too much of people. Know that every one of us has his or her place in the world; every quality is needed and there is a place for everyone and everything.

If we stop criticism concerning others, within ourselves, we are on our way. We have taken one of the first steps toward letting go of tension and working toward relaxation. We must do away with harmful comparison. Many people cannot help themselves and we should be tolerant of all things and all people. We need not necessarily accept all things, but we must learn to tolerate them if we desire to move forward toward relaxation. Only through understanding will we know how to think and know how the other person thinks. This is extremely important if we wish to get along with one another. Always make allowances for that which we do not understand in the other fellow. Many are misfits in their work but are forced on because of circumstances beyond their control and this means high tension. It is necessary then for them to find a hobby through which to release this tension.

IN NOTHING BE ANXIOUS

If you develop your spiritual philosophy constantly you will find freedom; your spiritual philosophy acts as a balance. We are told, "In nothing be anxious," yet anxiety is one of our chief difficulties. We are anxious about our business; the very food our bodies need; our family and our friends. Can we not KNOW that He who knows when the sparrow falls, certainly knows our needs too?

The greatest commandment is, "Love ye one another." Do We? Ask yourself: Am I not a little jealous of another person? Do I covet his job? His possessions? Could any of us be nailed to the cross and say, "Forgive them for they know not what they do?" "Could I go through a real ordeal, knowing someone else was responsible for it, without becoming agitated and upset? Am I truly thankful? How thankful am I?" Just saying, "Thank you, Father," will bring relaxation.

In working out your disease problems, you usually come to the place where you are tired of disease and then you start seeking a cure. In seeking a cure, I feel the first thing you will have to do is seek enlightenment. When I say, "seek enlightenment," I mean you must arrive at a point where you realize it is in your own habits; your manner of living; your own thinking, eating, drinking; the way you look at people; the way you look at yourself, which is causing your tension. In order to have health, you must look at these from every angle.

One of the first things you must do is start a "conversion" job in your mind and body. You must seek a higher level on which to live. You must get away from the old; break the old cycle, and possibly, when you read some of my work on "breaking the cycle," you will learn that it is possible to let go of the old and accept the new. There is a gospel of the spirit. We hear about the gospel in church; there is also a gospel of good health that will bring peace to your soul and bring more light to the spirit.

WAKE UP WISELY

To relax the mind for daily activities, try to create the right world for you to work and live in at the beginning. "Wake up wisely." To wake up wisely, always see to it that the right side of the bed is the side you get out on. You know it is said that there is a right and a wrong side of the bed. It is very important to start right. What are you going to say when you meet a person? Are you going to say, "How are you?" so that things come back to you in the form of trouble? No! Insist that the world you live in be a comfortable one; a soothing one: a good one. Do not invite gossip. Do not talk about troubles. Do not allow anyone else to talk about their troubles to you, unless you are a "trouble shooter;" unless you are a "professional listener;" unless you are paid to do that job and you have no way of getting out of it. There are lawyers to take care of money problems, suits, fights and arguments. You need not take care of these. There are times in your family life, when you should discuss these things, but nine times out of ten, everyone would be better off if he did not try to take on all the troubles of his neighborhood or of humanity in general.

Do not discuss your disease problem; discuss only the joys there are to be had in the world, upliftment. Work for the higher good of man, for we find that in sorrow and regret, remorse, illness, disease, hospitals, doctors, we have negative thoughts and attitudes, and in these thoughts we ruin our health.

When you meet others, immediately tell them how you are, so that you can bring out the best in them. People are not trained in the art of suggestion, these days, and as I have said before, suggestion makes its mark, so make sure that you bring out the best you know is in every person. If you bring out the best in the other person, you are serving him the best way he can be served, while you serve yourself as well.

When you say, "I feel wonderful," you are suggesting to others that they feel wonderful too, but if they tell you about their headache before you even say a word, they are suggesting, that you talk about your own headache. Instead of joy existing and a world of peace and harmony, we have two headaches trying to get along together. It reminds me of a little story I heard one time, how two "peeves" tried to get along in the same "pod." They didn't!

DO YOUR WORDS SING THEMSELVES INTO THE HEART?

Every word carries a vibratory action. It has been found that hate can actually destroy health, and that all the things which go with hate can destroy both the mind and the body. Words which include fear, resentment, resistance, harshness, create a vibratory force that is difficult to handle. We should train ourselves in a good philosophy and in the use of better, brighter words.

We must consistently train and educate ourselves to pick out joy and all that it means, peace and calmness. Reach for harmony and calm, soothing spirit. Realize that words which make up your world are found in our companions and in our occupations. These are the things that determine whether you are living in a healthy state of mind or in an ill state of mind.

RELAX TO COMBAT TENSION

To overcome tension, we must cultivate peace of mind and calmness in our mental processes. Relaxation will restore you to health and overcome tenseness, the cause of innumerable diseases.

"If you lose your money, you have lost something; If you lose your health, you have lost much; But if you lose your peace of mind, you have lost everything."

My job is to awaken you and get you to see that there is a better way to live than you are living. I know that many people have obtained more relaxation from the fact that they can now say, "Now I know. Now I see. Now things are better. Now I am on my way."

Having found a way to these accomplishments can bring relaxation to one who had been frustrated and did not know what to do about it. That person who is continually saying, "I wish I could find help, but I do not know where to go," is the person who is just wringing his hands and adding misery to misery; he has no relaxation in either mind or body.

Most of us live until we come to a place where the only one who can take care of the problem we face, seems to be a judge or the doctor. It seems that we always have to have someone take care of our problems after we create them. Very few people find the way of living that can keep them out of trouble.

Meditation brings relaxation more than anything else. Be honest with yourself in that "quiet time" we have spoken of. Take a moment to see that all is well; say to yourself, "All is well." No matter how much disturbance there is in the world, we should not allow ourselves to become disturbed too. If we are going to make a change in the world, someone must be less disturbed; someone must take control by having control. If we go to pieces because the world seems to be falling to pieces, we are going to save none of it, nor will the world be any better for our having lived in it. We have a definite job to do and that is to elevate ourselves to the place where we realize that peace and harmony and good will toward our fellowmen does exist.

While I was in Switzerland, I learned of a wonderful group called the M.R.A. Group. They have what is called the "Quiet Time," their meditation moments when they are looking toward the higher good for man. This good can work out for an individual or for a nation; it makes no difference because we know that the nation is made up of individuals.

This "Quiet Time" is necessary in our lives. The person who does not have a quiet time for recuperation, a quiet time for meditation, a quiet time to go into himself, will become bewildered or "rattled" and remain upset. We must have the opposite of worldly affairs in order to get in touch with the Godly affairs. There is a chamber within you in which you have this "quiet time". You have heard of those who do things on "Q.T." Well, the letters mean "Quiet Time", and if we can realize that we can do good on the "Q.T." as well as harm, we will most certainly accomplish the good and not the bad.

The person who "lets go and lets God", is allowing perfection to express itself. If we take upon ourselves that which we want to do, in most cases we are not letting God do it. When we are doing the Godly thing, we are dealing with the unchangeable factors in life, the highest factors. If we allow a Godly expression to take place at all times and forget our own will, a state of habitual peace will exist. No harm will ever rebound to ourselves and no harm will be done to the other person.

When it is said that we live "in the world but are not of it", this means that we do not live in this world of strife and fear, but in one of peace. Today you choose the direction in which you go. You either stand with God or you stand alone.

WHEN WE COME TO THE END OF A PERFECT DAY

As we go through life, we should find that we have built up things which add to our enjoyment. We take one picture after another of each moment we live, and as we recall them, these pictures of past moments should be pleasant, relaxing and enjoyable to us. What kind of an album are we assembling?

I say very sincerely that unless you have built up an album of beautiful pictures as you have gone through life, you cannot expect to have a beautiful ending. As we watch the sky and see the end of the day in a glorious sunset, we should also see these beautiful experiences colored in beauty and our album should mean a great deal to us. We may look at the sunset and realize that it means the end of us, but that which goes before a sunrise or a sunset could just as well be something better for us.

I look at some people who do nothing but "chase after the dollar" and my heart goes out to them. They never take time out for happiness, to go boating or to see a sunset or to think about a beautiful sunset. There should be a sunset for everyone and it can be a beautiful sunset, or it can be one with a very unhappy significance.

While lecturing at the Edgewater Beach Hotel in Chicago some time ago, the following was brought out to me. We had a group there, particularly interested in health. I was telling them how to achieve success through health and told them that the most important thing in this health work is to remember not to have a full stomach on leaving the table, but to leave the table with a stomach that feels "just comfortable," and I stressed that peace of mind also was very important to success.

I was then told that at this same Edgewater Beach Hotel, back in 1923, a group of the worlds' "most successful" financiers and leaders had met. The president of the largest independent steel company was there; also, the president of the largest utility company; the greatest wheat speculator; the president of the New York Stock Exchange; a member of the President's cabinet was there, as also was the "greatest bear on Wall Street." The president of the bank of International Settlements was there and the head of the world's greatest monopoly. Collectively, these great men controlled more wealth than there was in the United States Treasury. Their success stories were carried through the newspapers and magazines of the nation. These men were praised and lauded as examples for the youth of our nation to follow.

Let us follow through and see what happened to these "success" men twenty-five years later. The president of the largest independent steel company, Charles Schwab, was living on borrowed money, and did so the last five years of his life. He died broke.

The greatest wheat speculator, Arthur Cutten, died abroad, insolvent. The president of the New York Stock Exchange, Richard Whitney, served a term in Sing Sing. The member of the President's cabinet, Albert Fall, was pardoned from prison so that he might die at home.

The greatest "bear in Wall Street", Jesse Livermore, committed suicide. The president of the Bank of International Settlements, Leon Kreuger, committed suicide.

All of these men were successful in the eyes of the world and yet we find they all died a miserable death. Is that the price of "success", or what they call "good living"? Did they leave a "relaxed life, a happy life, a healthful life"? These are questions you will have to answer for yourselves.

Every human being is a child of God. We live in a beneficent order and only good can come to us when we live and observe spiritual laws which are also Nature's laws.

"He will sustain thee, be not weary in well doing." Total responsibility does not rest with man. It is in God's hands. Mind and body of man is as a great transformer, taking the energy and intelligence of the Divine and stepping them down to a vibratory rate which can be used by man for his perfect health and attainment. By yourself you can do nothing. "It is the Father that dwelleth in me; He doeth the work," said Jesus the Christ. But we have to "let" Him.

Relaxation is of the spirit as well as of the body and mind and the "letting go" to calmness originates in pure spirit and communicates to mind and body "Be still and know."

A calm attitude is against chaos which plunges man into tension and impatience. Unless we realize that the spiritual flows through all physical things, we cannot understand the Godly things which make for good health. Through a right spiritual attitude of tranquility, fretting, stewing and sorrowing will become unnecessary and will cease to interfere with good health.

"Let go and let God". The more we learn about ourselves the more tolerant we are of the other fellow.

"God grant me serenity to accept things I cannot change, courage to change the things I can, and wisdom to know the difference."

Thoughts impinge upon your consciousness from the vast storehouse of intelligence in space. Know positively that Good lies ahead of you if you would keep calm and poised. What you out picture manifests in your world, so be careful that only constructive, positive thoughts go out to return to you in health. Think only constructive, blessing thoughts; balance your diet; breathe deeply of fresh, clean air, and let sunlight flood into your organisms if you would have abundant health and fine understanding.

The opposite of dis-ease is ease. The opposite of tension is relaxation. If we do as David said: "Use your brain to forget with", relaxation is on its way. Relaxation, rest, sane living and laughter spell health and a good life.

CONSIDER THE ESSENES

Consider the ancient religion sect, the Essenes, who dwelt along the shore of the Red Sea. It is reported that Jesus the Christ was a member of the Essenes. If humanity would model its respective lives on the pattern adopted and set down by these people, healing and perfect health would be general. Tension of mind and body would be replaced by harmony of the cells and synchronization of the organs.

The Essenes were healers of marked ability. They went about teaching people how to live in accordance with the rhythm of the universe so that good health would be a permanent blessing. To establish health in their minds and bodies, they went "within" to find inner peace. In contacting this eternal inner peace, the peace that "passeth understanding," they sought to be at peace with all their neighbors, hostile or friendly, known or unknown, to the end that complete harmony should function on the earth.

One day of each week was set aside by the Essenes for meditation on peace with neighbors. They found that they had to get along together, for this is the highest virtue tending toward spirituality. To do so, they had to purge from their consciousness all jealousies, all prejudices, all barriers of race, creed or color. They wanted to hasten the day when men would be proud to belong to the human race with its Divine heritage.

Another day of the week, they set aside for meditation upon peace among members of their families. They learned and practiced tolerance of the other person and his actions and views, on the premise that each human soul was doing the best he or she could at the level of his development where he then stood, and therefore no blame should be attached.

One day of the week was devoted to establishing peace with knowledge and culture. And on the last day of the week, the Essenes, through deep meditation, sought peace that comes from Wisdom and the Heavenly Father. This highly spiritual sect sought a peaceful life and their manner of living set them apart from most of humanity. They were readily recognized everywhere in their communities by their actions of Love. These Essenes knew the value of water in healing and in maintaining perfect health.

They also knew about clay packs and water packs and their high value in healing. They followed the pattern set by Jesus when he used clay upon the eyes of the blind man.

If we will work toward coming into harmony with those about us, tension will go, ill health will be replaced by mental and physical wellbeing if we are in harmony. We give and take. This harmony even applies to the soil in which is grown the fruits and vegetables; indeed, all things for man's maintenance and good. Unless we give back to the soil the nutriment which we now take from it, we shall starve in the midst of plenty, for a willful waste will make a woeful want.

If you should ask me for some magic formula to banish tension and ill health, I would advise "balanced living, sane food selection and preparation, natural live foods, sunshine and fresh air and rhythmic breathing, rest and sleep, the use of real power of suggestion, and a calm attitude of mind."

EXERCISES

1. Sit in a chair, straight backed and of comfortable height, feet flat on the floor, hands on knees, palms upward. Inhale six times; one long breath, then exhale.

A person who knows how to relax will breathe very slowly. A mouse breathes 100 times a minute. An elephant breathes three to six times a minute. Long-lived animals are those which take long, slow breaths. If you are impatient, your breath comes and goes quickly. If you excite the heart, you excite the breath. Fear causes you to breathe faster. Your mental attitude determines how you breathe.

2. Before going to sleep, lie flat on your back, either on the floor or in bed. Lift the hands, relax and let go. Lift the forearms, relax and let go. And I mean limp like, just like a rag doll. Lift up the legs, relax and let go. Lift the head, relax and let go. Lift up the body from the waist, then lower. Let the floor or bed hold you, completely relaxed. Lie on your side, let go of your arms. Tell your whole body to "relax and let go." Let go in all directions.

3. Stand erect, shake hands, letting them shake limply, let go. Then arms. Let the head go forward and backward, letting go at the neck.

4. Raise hands above your head. Claw your hands; do not clench. A closed hand cannot receive anything. With clawed hands and upraised arms, inhale, and pull as if chinning yourself on a bar; exhale, relax and let go.

5. Stretch arms forward, hands clasped; pull with inhalation; relax with exhalation. Up then down, then left to right, as if one arm is pulling against the other. Then clasp hands behind back and try to push backward.

6. Stand erect; take in breath slowly through nostrils; raise arms while breathing and holding this thought. "Peace and harmony." Exhale and let body bend forward to waist, completely relaxed again, like a rag doll. Slowly resume standing position. Think tall. Feel tall.

Serenity of mind is a big factor in maintaining good health. This serenity comes when you know your close relationship with the ruling power of the universe; that His power is yours to use for Good.

OTHER BOOKLETS BY DR. JENSEN

1. HOW TO ENJOY BETTER HEALTH FROM NATURAL REMEDIES

2. HOW TO RELAX AND RELIEVE TENSION

3. HOW TO REVITALIZE YOUR GLANDS

4. A NEW SLANT ON HEALTH AND BEAUTY—SLANT BOARD

5. A HEALTH PATTERN TO LIVE BY

6. HOW TO BUILD A BETTER BODY FROM YOUR KITCHEN

7. HOW THE BREATH OF LIVE SUSTAINS YOU

8. PHYSICAL, MENTAL AND SPIRITUAL BALANCE

9. DEVELOPING INWARD CALM

10. THE NEED FOR A NEW ATTITUDE

11. THE HEART OF CIRCULATORY SYSTEM

12. THREE STEPS TO THE HIGHER LIFE (Part I)

13. THREE STEPS TO THE HIGHER LIFE (Part II)

14. THREE STEPS TO THE HIGHER LIFE (Part III)

15. HEALTH FOR OUR CHILDREN

16. SPECIAL FOODS FOR SPECIAL NEEDS

17. LETS BEGIN AT THE BEGINNING

18. YOUR LOVE LIFE

19. INTESTINAL DISORDERS & FASTING & ELIMINATIVE DIETS

20. VOL. I — SECRETS I CAN SHARE WITH YOU

21. VOL. 11 — MORE SECRETS I CAN SHARE WITH YOU

MEET THE ORIGINAL AUTHOR

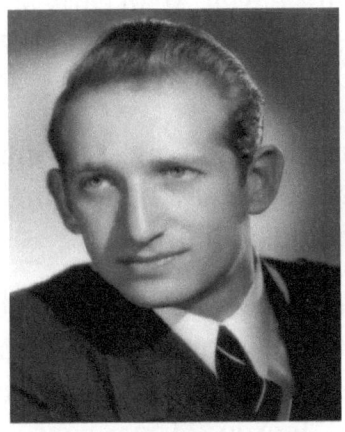

(From the back of the booklet)

Bernard Jensen, D.C, N.D., Nutritionist of Los Angeles, Calif. Born in Stockton, Calif, in 1908.

Possessing a convincing philosophy that would credit much older practitioners, Bernard Jensen, D.C, Lecturer and Teacher of Right Living, acquired from the beginning of his studies the vision "that Nature does all the healing." He believes doctors can only work with natural laws. His work is sane, up-to-date, practical and teaches a balanced "how-to-live" regime.

At only 18, Dr. Jensen began studies with the West Coast Chiropractic College, Oakland, Calif. At 21 he began his practice of chiropractic in that city and has been practicing that science ever since. Widely traveled, he has been honored with post-graduate degrees from the National College in Chicago and the American School of Naturopathy, New York. He studied methods of the Battle Creek Sanitarium, of Tilden's School of Fasting in Denver. At an early age he was teaching his "How-to-live" methods to professional groups.

For 50 years. Dr. Jensen has led a most strenuous life, lecturing, radio broadcasting and directing his own health center in Escondido, California.

His current plans include Radio and TV guest appearances, a nationwide tour, and more contributions to Iridology and color, with new works planned in both areas. Dr. Jensen's The Science and Practice of Iridology has brought him international acclaim and is currently being translated into Spanish. Nine more books are in various stages of production, including his spiritual masterpiece. Arise and Shine, and color book.

HIDDEN VALLEY HEALTH RANCH

Comfortable Accommodations

The accommodations are gaily decorated and furnished with every comfort – restful beds, spacious closets and individually controlled heat. Each room will assure you a pleasant stay and a full night's sleep every night. Every attempt is made to make you as comfortable as possible. Accommodations are available at various rates to suit you.

Experience a new way of life, a non-demanding, relaxing, revitalizing way of living. Nestled in rolling country and continually blessed by pure fresh air, the ranch stretches over 200 acres of nature's artistry.

Your Hidden Valley vacation, or weekend may well become a recurring part of your recreational plans. It is here that we make the best use of nature...organically grown food, exercise, pure water and the right mental attitude all contribute to a vacation of unsurpassed value. Sun worshippers will enjoy the pool area or a leisurely walk around the ranch and hills can satisfy the desires of strollers, walkers or hardy hikers.

ABOUT THE AUTHOR

Jon Jensen, Iridologist, CMH, has been involved in holistic health for over 30 years with experience in Iridology, nutrition, and personal self-development. Jon started taking classes in Iridology and nutrition from his grandfather, the late Dr. Bernard Jensen in 1980. Dr. Bernard Jensen is generally regarded throughout North America as the forefather of Iridology. Jon filled numerous roles over the years and participated in his grandfather's many classes and projects. Jon was involved in research for his grandfather's books, helping to pioneer a new way of iris analysis using the computer, and assisting with seminars.

In 1995 Jon stayed by his grandfather's side after Dr. Bernard Jensen became paralyzed from the waist down from a car accident. Jon was an integral part of his grandfather's plan to walk again, treating the whole person; body, mind, and spirit and being a part of every aspect of what the doctors called a "Miracle"—as his grandfather walked again on his own.

After his grandfather's recovery, Jon shifted his attention to additional training by taking classes with some of the prominent leaders in the fields of Sclerology with Dr. Leonard Mehlmauer, Rayid (emotional iridology) with Denny Johnson, European based integrated iridology with Dr. Ellen Tart-Jensen as well as animal iridology with Dr. Mercedes Colburn. Jon attended Kalos© classes with Dr. Valerie Seeman-Gersch learning about Transformational Healing methods.

Jon was President of the Escondido Chapter of Chamber Toastmasters and enjoys speaking to groups.

Jon wrote an article for The Price-Pottenger Nutrition Foundation Journal on Animal Iridology/Nutrition. Jon has given presentations at: Holistic Health Fairs/Expo's, Herb Shops, and Health Food Stores.

Jon is currently Executive Director at the "Live Pure Kids" foundation in Arizona. Jon works closely with Gavin Tucker the President/Founder, and Jackie Morales, Vice President. The foundation is dedicated to educating the next generation on how to live a healthy lifestyle by encompassing a holistic approach to life through balancing the mind, body and spirit. www.livepurekids.com

Jon recently published a nutrition book called, "A Simple Guide to Healthy Living" and is available for purchase on Amazon.

For more information Jon can be found at www.jensenholistichealth.com or www.bernardjensen.org

www.ingramcontent.com/pod-product-compliance
Lightning Source LLC
Chambersburg PA
CBHW021254280526
45784CB00005B/2364